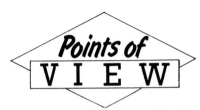

Points of VIEW

·M·E·D·I·C·A·L·
·E·T·H·I·C·S·

Jenny Bryan

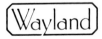

Points of View

Advertising
Alcohol
Animal Rights
Apartheid
Censorship
Divorce
Drugs

Medical Ethics
Northern Ireland
Nuclear Weapons
Racism
Sexuality
Smoking
Terrorism

Front cover: *A premature baby is cared for in a high technology incubator. From our first breath to our last, we may need medical help — the ethical issues raised by medicine affect us all.*

Excerpt from *In the Company of Others*, copyright © 1982 by Jory Graham, reprinted by permission of Harcourt Brace Jovanovich, Inc.

Editor: William Wharfe
Designer: David Armitage

First published in 1989 by
Wayland (Publishers) Limited
61 Western Road, Hove
East Sussex BN3 1JD, England

©Copyright 1989 Wayland (Publishers) Limited

British Library Cataloguing in Publication Data
Bryan, Jenny
    Medical ethics. — (Points of view)
    1. Medicine. Ethical aspects
    I. Title   II. Series
    174'.2

ISBN 1-85210-801-0

Phototypeset by Direct Image Photosetting Ltd,
Hove, East Sussex, England.
Printed in Italy by G. Canale & C.S.p.A., Turin
Bound in France by A.G.M.

Contents

Introduction

> I swear by Apollo the physician, and Aesculapius and Health, and All-heal, and all the gods and goddesses, that . . . I will follow that system of regimen which, according to my ability and judgement, I consider for the benefit of my patients; and abstain from whatever is deleterious and mischievous. I will give no deadly medicine to anyone if asked, nor suggest any such counsel; and in like manner I will not give to a woman a pessary to produce abortion . . . Into whatever houses I enter, I will go into them for the benefit of the sick, and will abstain from every voluntary act of mischief and corruption; and, further, from the seduction of females, or males, or freemen or slaves. Whatever, in connection with my professional practice, or not in connection with it, I see or hear, in the life of men, which ought not to be spoken of abroad, I will not divulge, as reckoning that all such should be kept secret . . .

The above is an extract from the Hippocratic Oath — the earliest attempt to set out a code of ethics within which doctors should work. There have since been many changes and revisions.

Doctors all over the world, such as these pictured in Nairobi, Kenya, still take the Hippocratic Oath at the end of their medical training.

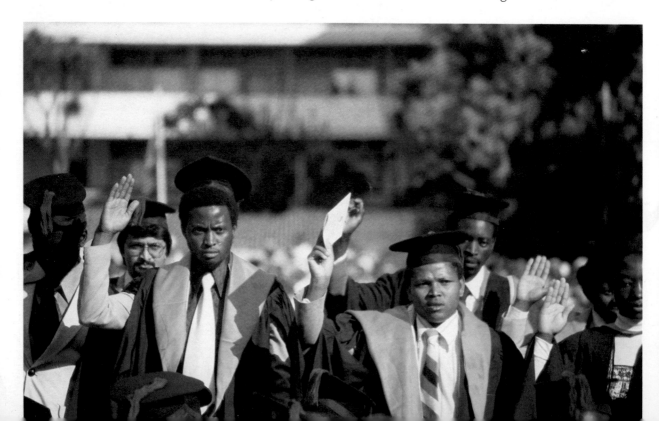

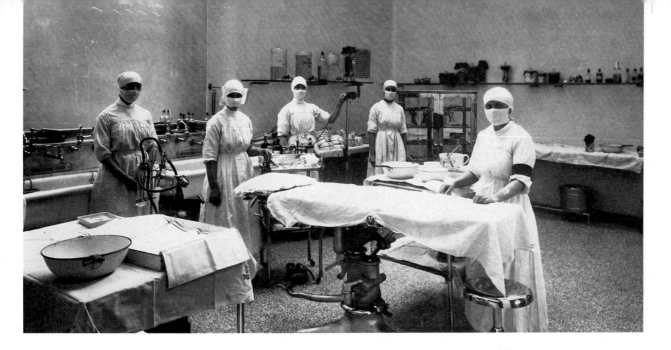

Today the list of duties of physicians to the sick outlined in the Declaration of Geneva is perhaps more appropriate:

> • A physician shall always bear in mind the obligation of preserving human life.

• A physician shall owe his patients complete loyalty and all the resources of his science. Whenever an examination or treatment is beyond the physician's capacity he should summon another physician who has the necessary ability.

• A physician shall preserve absolute confidentiality on all he knows about his patient even after the patient has died.

• A physician shall give emergency care as a humanitarian duty unless he is assured that others are willing and able to give such care.
(International Code of Medical Ethics, based on Declaration of Geneva, World Medical Association.)

Medicine has, of course, moved on too; what doctors see as doing their best for their patient is different today from what it was just a decade ago. Where once the emphasis was on prolonging life at all costs, doctors now talk of the importance of improving the quality of life.

The exciting but expensive advances in the diagnosis and treatment of disease have brought with them new and more complex ethical dilemmas for today's medical profession. Now, doctors must decide whether they *can* treat their patients, whether they *should* treat them and, not least, if society is able and willing to pay.

An operating theatre at St Bartholomew's Hospital, London, in 1920. Medical advances since then have vastly improved the success rate of operations, but in some cases they have also caused ethical dilemmas.

2

Whose body is it anyway?

What should we reasonably expect our doctor to tell us about our illness and any proposed treatment? Some people want to know more than others and a few would prefer to leave all the decisions to their doctor. No medical treatment is without risk; all drugs, for example, have unwanted as well as beneficial effects and many operations involve some risk of trauma to the patient.

For example, in 1974 an elderly British woman, Mrs Amy Sidaway, had an operation to relieve severe pain in her neck and shoulder. There were serious complications and she was left partially paralysed. Mrs Sidaway sued her health authority for damages of £67,500 on the grounds that she had not been sufficiently warned of the risk of spinal damage – a risk that had been estimated at between one and two per cent – before she gave her written consent to surgery. When her case finally went to court in 1984 her claim was dismissed on the grounds that she was told as much as would have been accepted as proper by a responsible body of skilled and experienced neuro-surgeons.

How difficult is it for doctors to assess how much information we want and need in order to consent to treatment?

__Below__ A sign in India advertising the benefits of vaccination. Successful mass immunization relies on people voluntarily consenting to being vaccinated. How much should they be told about the risks involved?

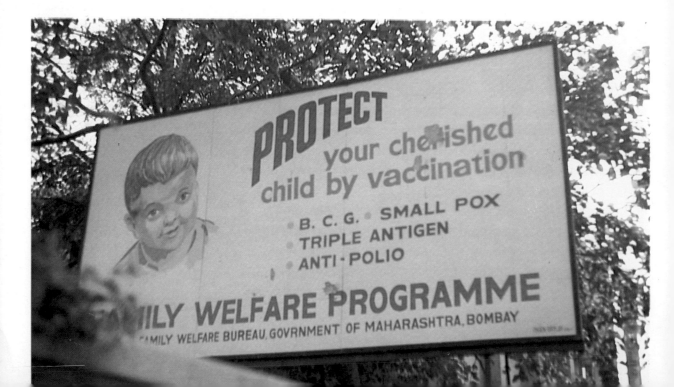

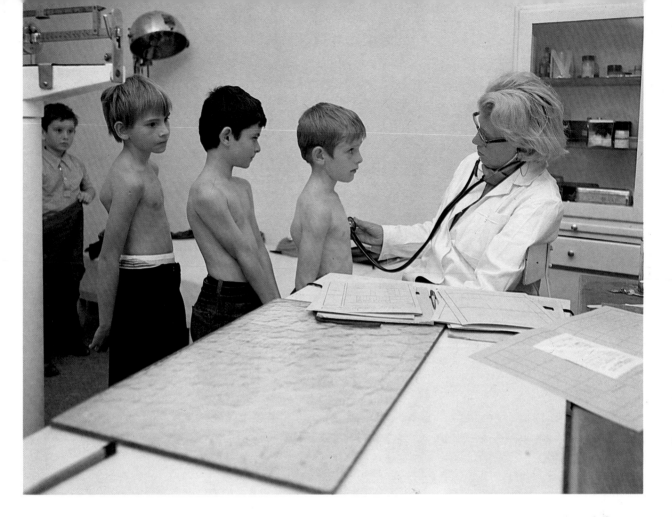

Above *A doctor with some young patients: how much should she explain about the treatment she prescribes?*

> As a doctrine and as a practical reality, informed consent is neither so complicated nor so difficult as doctors and lawyers would make it, nor is there any good reason for the extended medical debates it engenders. At its core, it is respect for the patient as an individual, not a defence against the possibility of a later malpractice suit. (Jory Graham, *In the Company of Others.*)

In the USA, a Patients' Bill of Rights has been drawn up to set out precisely what patients should demand:

> - The patient has the right to informed participation in all decisions involving his health care programme.
> - The patient has a right to know what research and experimental protocols are being used.
> - The patient has a right to a clear, concise explanation of all proposed procedures in layman's terms, including the possibilities of any risk of mortality, of serious side effects, problems relating to recuperation, and probability of success. (George J. Annas, *The Rights of Hospital Patients: the Basic ACLU Guide to a Hospital Patient's Rights,* 1976.)

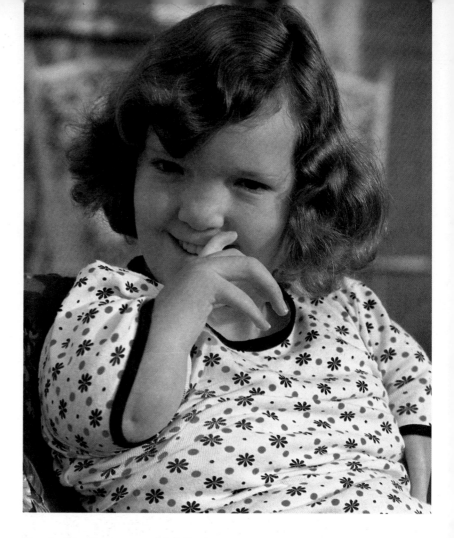

The dangers of the drug thalidomide were not known during the early 1960s, and many children were born with deformed arms and legs after their mothers had taken the drug during pregnancy.

But is this always possible? Each year, thousands of patients are asked to take part in studies of new treatments which may or may not help them. Often, the doctors themselves are unaware of the possible risks and benefits.

> The trouble with informed consent is that it is not educated consent . . . the chances are remote that the subject really understands what he has consented to – in the sense that the responsible medical investigator understands the goals, nature and hazards of his study. How can the layman comprehend the importance of his perhaps not receiving, as determined by the luck of the draw, the highly touted new treatment that his room-mate will get? How can he appreciate the sensation of living for days with a multi-lumen intestinal tube passing through his mouth and pharynx? How can he interpret the information that an intravascular catheter and radiopaque dye injection have an 0.01 per cent probability of leading to a dangerous thrombosis or cardiac arrhythmia?

What should I ask?
1 What will happen in this test/treatment?
2 Why do you think I should have it?
3 What are the likely risks, both immediately and over the next few months or years?
4 What are the alternatives?

Nor can the information given to the experimental subject be in any sense totally complete. It would be impractical and probably unethical for the investigator to present the nearly endless list of all possible contingencies; in fact, he may not himself be aware of every untoward thing that might happen. (Franz Ingelfinger, *New England Journal of Medicine*, 31 August, 1972.)

Getting informed consent from the mentally ill or senile is especially difficult. Doctors operate within guidelines laid down by their professional organizations:

> When an adult is mentally incapable of giving valid consent, e.g. by reason of mental illness, serious subnormality or senility, the doctor must decide, as in any other case, what is in the best interests of the patient. No other individual, unless duly appointed as a guardian, has legal authority to consent to treatment on the patient's behalf. (British Medical Association, *Philosophy and Practice of Medical Ethics.*)

But it may be difficult to judge whether someone who is mentally ill is refusing treatment because he or she does not understand what is involved or because they, like anyone else, are worried about the risks they face.

If mentally ill people — depicted here in the film Frances *— are incapable of giving valid consent to treatment, who should make the decision for them?*

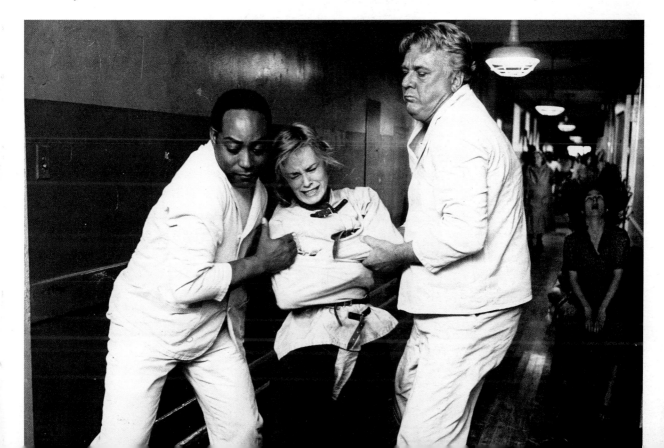

> Although some of these [mentally ill] patients may be incapable of looking after themselves or their affairs, they may be *intermittently* competent to give consent. Some of the time they may be as lucid and aware as any sane person and certainly capable of understanding that their consent is needed and what it implies . . . A mental patient who objects to a course of electroconvulsive therapy (ECT), for instance, may be no more 'irrational' than a cancer patient who refuses chemotherapy.

In both cases, the patient may be quite rationally questioning whether the effects of the treatment will improve the quality of her life as she sees it. (Carolyn Faulder, *Whose Body Is It?*)

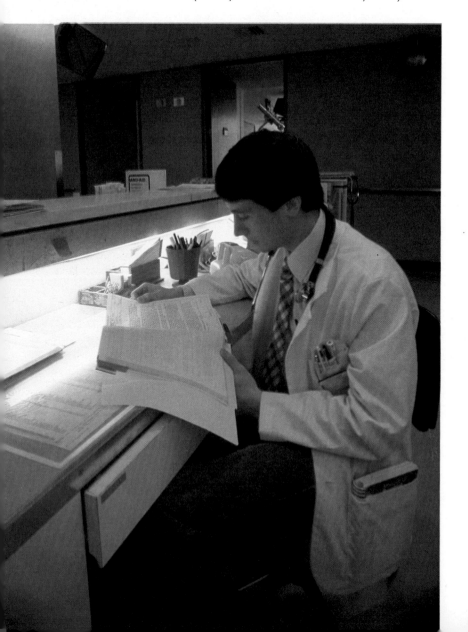

Left *A doctor in Greenwich Hospital, Connecticut, USA, consulting the medical records of one of his patients. Recently, some people have demanded to see their own records, but not all doctors are happy about having their comments revealed to their patients.*

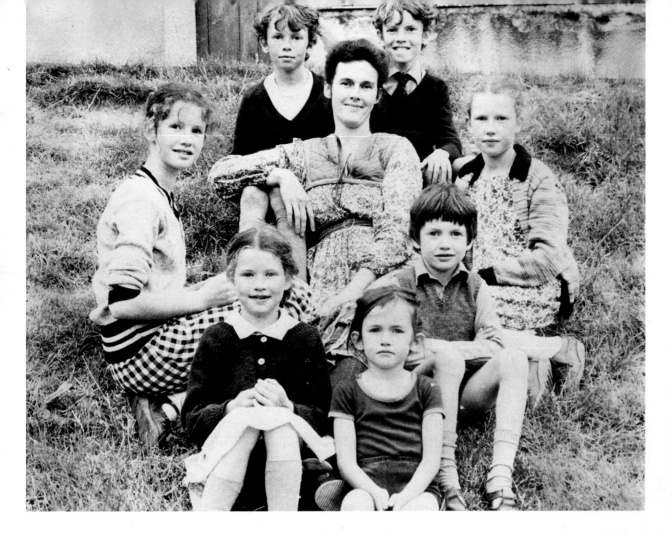

What about children? Who should make decisions about treatment for them? In the UK, the age of consent has been set at sixteen and parents or guardians generally take decisions about treatment for children below that age. Yet in a recent protracted legal battle *(Gillick versus West Norfolk and Wisbech AHA)* over the questions of whether doctors should be allowed to prescribe the contraceptive pill to girls under sixteen without their parents' consent, the judge pointed out:

> The fact that a child is under the age of sixteen does not mean automatically that she cannot give consent to any treatment. Whether or not a child is capable of giving the necessary consent will depend on the child's maturity and understanding and the nature of the consent which is required. The child must be capable of making a reasonable assessment of the advantages and disadvantages of the treatment proposed, so the consent if given can be properly and fairly described as a true consent. *(Gillick v. West Norfolk and Wisbech AHA.)*

Above *Victoria Gillick with seven of her ten children. In Britain, in 1985, she lost her fight to prevent children under sixteen being prescribed contraceptives without the consent of their parents.*

A new-born baby about to be weighed. An ethical problem has arisen in recent years with some women claiming that they have the right to give birth in their own home, despite regulations in some countries that state that they must go into hospital.

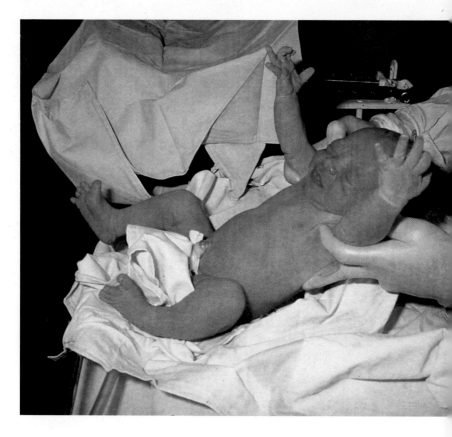

1   Imagine you are going into hospital to have your tonsils out. What would you ask your doctor about the operation and your treatment afterwards?

2   Doctors in the UK may now prescribe the contraceptive pill to a girl under sixteen without her parents' consent only if they are sure that she:

a) fully understands the advice she is being given
b) cannot be persuaded that her parents should be told
c) is likely to begin or continue having sexual intercourse with or without contraception
d) will suffer mentally or physically unless she receives contraceptive advice, and that it is in her best interests to receive treatment.

What do you think of these guidelines? Are they too strict on doctors or on teenage girls? At what age and under what circumstances do you think contraceptive advice and treatment should be available to young people? Explain your reasons.

There is no doubt that, at least in Western countries, patients are being given more information about their health. But there are now fears that doctors will use the practice of giving out information about treatment merely as a way of protecting themselves against legal action if something goes wrong. People worry that if a doctor has warned them of all the potential risks involved in treatment, then they will not be able to hold him or her responsible if something does go wrong.

In the UK and USA, patients must prove that a doctor, hospital or health authority has been at fault or negligent in the treatment given. In Sweden and New Zealand there is no need to prove who is to blame, only that damage has been done. Compensation is then paid out of a central insurance fund. In the USA, where levels of compensation are the highest in the world, lawyers are paid a percentage of the winnings, so it is in their interests to win the highest possible amount of financial compensation for their clients. There is a continuing and often fierce debate in many countries about what is the best way of making sure that both patient and doctor are treated fairly.

3

The right to end a life

> The direct interruption of the generative process already begun, and, above all, directly willed and procured abortion, even if for therapeutic reasons, are to be absolutely excluded as licit [lawful] means of regulating birth. (Papal encyclical, *Humanae Vitae*, 1968.)

There is no doubting the Roman Catholic Church's stand on abortion, the above quotation makes that very clear — under all circumstances, it is morally wrong. But abortion is practised legally or illegally throughout the world and has been for centuries. In countries such as the UK, USA and Australia, where it is legal, the question is not so much whether abortion is right or wrong, but under what circumstances it is justified. In many Eastern European Communist countries abortion is seen as a substitute for contraception.

> Anthropological and archaeological evidence shows that abortions have been performed for millennia. They are accepted because most societies hold the rights of pregnant women above those of a fetus without personhood . . . Christian philosophers thought that personhood began at quickening [see glossary], a poorly defined but convenient time.

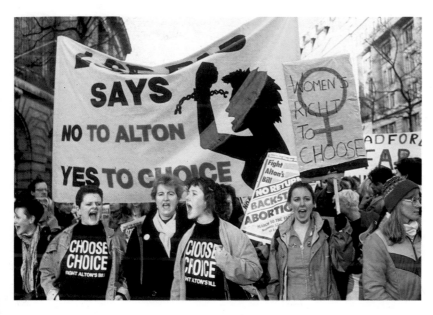

A demonstration in London, in 1988, against legislation proposed by British MP John Alton to tighten the conditions under which a legal abortion could be performed.

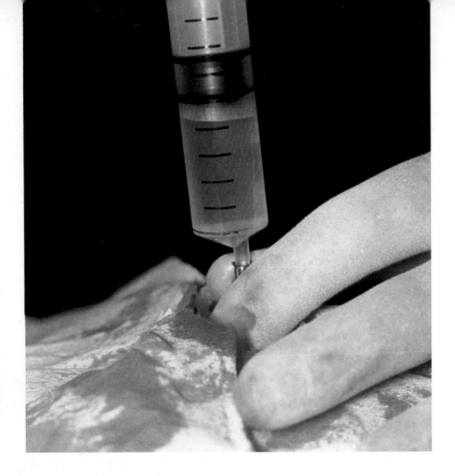

New York State restricted execution of pregnant women to those who had not felt fetal movement. The Talmud [Jewish Law] permits child destruction to save the mother until the birth of the head. Some philosophers and societies think that personhood is achieved only after birth. (Dr Peter Bromwich, *British Medical Journal*, 28 February, 1987.)

Medical advances in the last decade have meant that babies born as early as 23 weeks can now survive and this has called into question the time limits put on abortion in countries where the procedure is legal. But the results of many of the tests for abnormal babies, which parents may decide to terminate, are frequently not available until after 18-20 weeks of pregnancy. So demands to reduce the time limit for abortion could put these tests in jeopardy or at least give the parents very little time in which to make a major decision.

> The great bugaboo of the anti-abortion campaign has always been that of the late termination, when babies cry before being tossed into the incinerator. Feminists impale themselves on the insistence that women should have the right to kill the fetus at any stage in the pregnancy while anti-abortionists speak

Abortion limits

Abortion is illegal only in Ireland, Portugal and parts of South America. In the UK it is legal on physical or mental grounds up to the twenty-eighth week of pregnancy. In the USA precise limits vary from state to state but, in general, abortion is available on request during the first trimester (up to 3 months) of pregnancy, on medical grounds during the second trimester (4-6 months) and, after that, only if the mother's life is in danger.

of all pregnancy termination as if it was third-trimester [after six months] abortion. There is something ghoulish in this fixation on abortion after quickening and something downright absurd in the pretension that all fetuses, whether ten days old or ten weeks old or twenty weeks old, are the same sort of thing. (Germaine Greer, *Sex and Destiny – the Politics of Human Fertility*, 1984.)

Various proposals for time limits on abortion have been made:

> What would seem logical, from the present standpoint, is a change in our present abortion law, so as to allow abortion on demand before the neural structures underlying consciousness have developed (say, within the first ten weeks) but imposing more stringent conditions thereafter. Clearly, also, one should set an earlier time limit for any abortion of a normal child, where the mother's life or physical health is not endangered by continued pregnancy, than applies at present, since babies have now been born alive a full five weeks before the present limit on abortions [28 weeks] . . . The present time limit could be retained, however, for abortions that were genuinely therapeutic [medically necessary], or proposed because of some grave and inoperable defect in the fetus . . . (Michael Lockwood, *Moral Dilemmas in Modern Medicine*, 1985.)

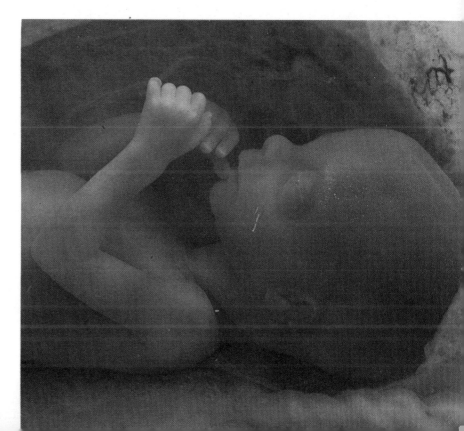

Right *The subject of the argument over abortion. A human fetus photographed twelve weeks after conception.*

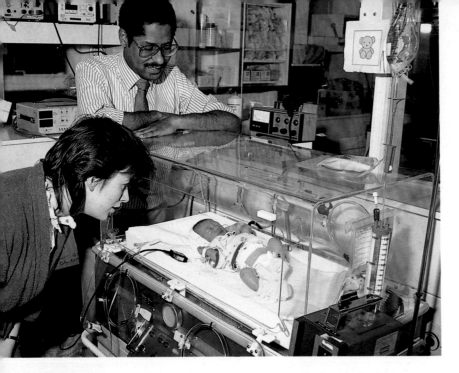

The ability to save very premature babies has brought other dilemmas. Although they can be kept alive where once they would have died, some will grow up physically or mentally handicapped. Should every effort be made to save them or should they be allowed to die?

> Once we accept that there are certain classes — i.e. unwanted unborn children, unwanted infants who are retarded or handicapped, etc. — whose lives are unworthy of legal protection, upon what moral high ground do we stand to decry when Dr Himmler slaps us on the back, and asks us if he can include Gypsies and Jews? (Patrick J. Buchanan, former aid to US President Richard Nixon and speech writer for former US President Ronald Reagan, quoted in *The End of Life* by James Rachels.)

The mention of 'Dr Himmler' refers ironically to the Nazi leader who, during the 1930s and 1940s, was in charge of a programme of mass execution of Jews and Gypsies. The author is suggesting that the euthanasia of severely handicapped infants is essentially the same as the Nazi's execution of people because of their race.

The above quotation is typical of the 'slippery slope' argument, which appears frequently in medical ethics; that is: if we allow one exception to our moral code, will this lead to other, less acceptable exceptions? Yet the problems of bringing up a severely handicapped child should not be underestimated and are probably best summed up by parents.

Ending life

Euthanasia — mercy killing — is illegal in all countries. But many countries have legal or ethical codes governing the circumstances under which life support machines may be turned off — and tests which must be performed to ensure that 'brain death' has occurred; that is: all functions of the brain have permanently and irreversibly ceased, whether or not the function of some organs, such as the heartbeat, have been maintained artificially.

There is a strong consumer lobby in favour of legalizing euthanasia in certain circumstances. In Holland, for example, where the law has turned a 'blind eye' to cases of euthanasia, an estimated 10,000 seriously ill or incurable patients each year persuade their doctor to help them die and a survey in one region showed that 80 per cent of doctors had direct experience of euthanasia.

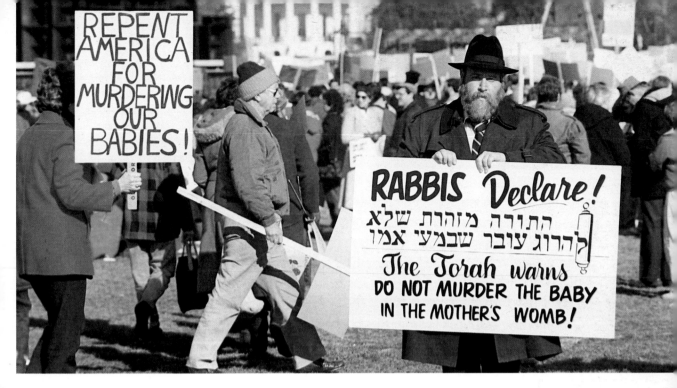

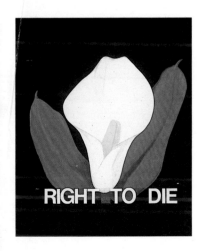

Above *The Roman Catholic Church is seen as the religion most firmly against abortion, but the Jewish community has also campaigned against it.*

Below *This is the logo for EXIT — the British organization which has campaigned for the legalization of euthanasia.*

> Oh if I could have got away with it I would have neglected him because I was so fed up and tired more than anything, so if I could have got away with it I would have neglected him. I'm sorry I didn't in a way. You've got to be honest — they are a tie for the rest of your life . . . there's not going to be any freedom at all.
>
> It's all right for those who've never had one to say, 'keep him alive'. On the surface things don't look any different, but in reality it's a continual strain. You don't show it outside. *(Parents and Mentally Handicapped Children, 1980.)*

If severely handicapped children are to be allowed to die, what of the argument for active euthanasia?

> If voluntary euthanasia were legalized, there is good reason to believe that at a later date another bill for compulsory euthanasia would be legalized. Once the respect for human life is so low that an innocent person may be killed directly even at his own request, compulsory euthanasia will necessarily be very near.
>
> This could lead easily to killing all incurable charity patients, the aged who are a public care, wounded soldiers, all deformed children, the mentally afflicted, and so on. Before long the danger would be at the door of every citizen. (Bishop Joseph V. Sullivan, *Beneficent Euthanasia*, 1975, edited by Martin Kohl.)

With very few exceptions the medical profession is united in its view.

> Where a terminally ill patient's coma is beyond doubt irreversible, and there are adequate safeguards to confirm the accuracy of the diagnosis, all means of life support may be discontinued. If death does not occur when life support systems are discontinued, the comfort and dignity of the patient should be maintained. (American Medical Association, *Principles of Medical Ethics*, 1982.)

The dilemma of whether anyone has the right to end a life, whether that is by refraining from giving care, or by actively killing, is not new. What has brought it to the fore is the increasing ability to save or to end life which advances in high technology medicine have brought with them. Perhaps, the last word should go to a Roman philosopher who lived nearly 2000 years ago, when life support was limited to food and drink.

> I will not relinquish old age if it leaves my better part intact. But if it begins to shake my mind, if it destroys my faculties one by one, if it leaves me not life but death . . . If I know that I must suffer without hope of relief I will depart not through fear of the pain but because it prevents all for which I would live. (Lucius Annaeus Seneca, 58th letter to Lucilius.)

1   List as many reasons as you can, both for and against legalized abortion. Do you think there should be a time limit on abortion? If so, why?
2   Do you know someone who has or has had a serious illness (such as AIDS, cancer, a heart attack or arthritis)? What sorts of problems have they had to face? What steps do you think could have been taken to help them cope better?

Left *Hungarian born novelist Arthur Koestler made a suicide pact with his wife. When he became very ill in 1983 they both killed themselves.*

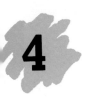

Animal experimentation

Each year millions of animals are used for laboratory experiments. The vast majority of those used are mice, rats, rabbits and guinea-pigs, but dogs, cats, fish and monkeys are also used. Most of the experiments are carried out by industrial companies to check the safety of commonly-used chemicals and medicines. University and hospital researchers also do a large number of experiments on animals in their search for new and better treatments for disease. In a significant number of cases, however, there is no obvious application for the research. Instead, there is the hope that such 'basic' research will ultimately lead to a medical breakthrough. But how far can these aspects of laboratory experimentation be justified? Are animal rights more important than scientific advancements?

> Relieving human need and suffering is an extremely urgent priority without which our species — and indeed the natural world as such — may not survive the century. Relative to this cause, that of animal welfare, though not unimportant, appears of considerably lower priority. Lamentably, it often seems that among the most vociferous [outspoken] proponents of animal welfare there is an abundance of concern for the plight of other species and very little for that of our own. (Michael Allen Fox, *The Case for Animal Experimentation,* 1986.)

Tight controls are kept on the type of experiments for which animals can be used — and on the conditions in which they are kept.

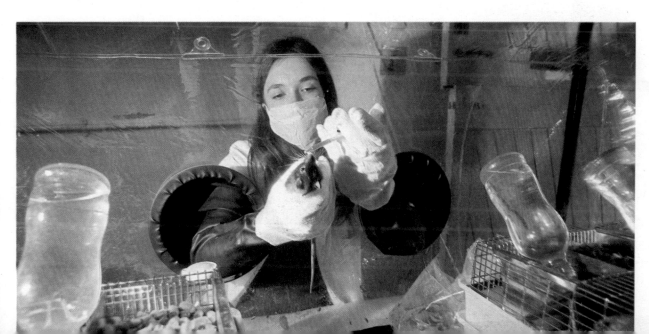

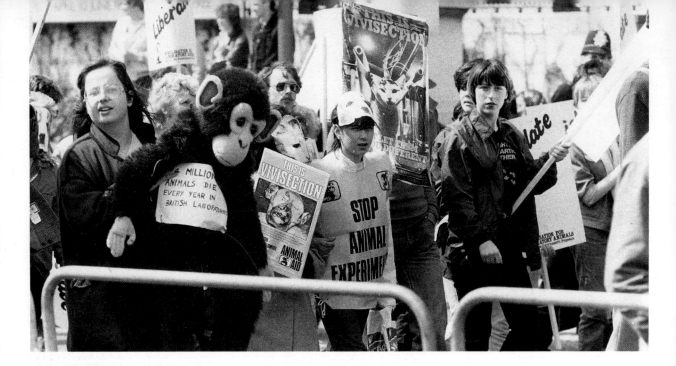

Some animal-rights campaigners became increasingly outspoken during the 1980s, sometimes also resorting to measures such as breaking into research units and releasing the animals kept for experiments.

> Of the 60 million animals used in US labs each year, only a small portion are involved in research into dread diseases such as cancer. Millions of animals die for such frivolous reasons as testing of new cosmetics, shampoos, household cleansers and radiator fluid when safe products already exist. (Lawrence Finsen, 'The Animal Rights People May Not Be So Misguided After All', *Los Angeles Times*, 3 June, 1985.)

In Western countries any chemical or medicine destined for human consumption must, by law, be thoroughly tested before it is marketed. Developing countries, which do not have the facilities or expertise to carry out such tests rely on the stamp of approval from countries such as the USA, UK and West Germany as a guarantee that a new product is safe. The final stage of this testing procedure involves human volunteers and patients, but before this can begin large numbers of animal experiments are carried out to try to ensure that a new product is not toxic. Is this really necessary?

> Consider the similarities between yourself and a mouse, what possible faith can you have that a drug that has been tested on animals will work for you? The fact is that animal experiments tell us about animals and not about people. They are irrelevant to humans and the results can prove to be dangerously misleading whilst many potentially useful drugs could also have been lost due to animal tests. (British Union for the Abolition of Vivisection, *Health with Humanity*, 1988.)

The end of LD-50

A major success story in controlling the need for animal experimentation has come with the dramatic reduction in recent years in the number of LD-50 (lethal dose – 50 per cent) tests on new drugs. To comply with government regulations throughout the world, it was previously necessary to identify the dose of any new drug which would kill 50 per cent of animals tested. Inevitably, this meant that large numbers of animals were killed. Scientific advances and pressure from researchers themselves have meant that the LD-50 test is no longer a routine requirement in many countries.

But, according to transplant pioneer Sir Roy Calne, the ability to cure most dangerous infections, to repair many heart defects and enable patients with kidney disease to lead normal lives are just three medical advances made possible solely by experiments on animals.

> If the public wishes to have such advantages of modern medicine as antibiotics and insulin, experiments on animals must be accepted. If you do not wish animals to be exploited then you must eschew all modern medical treatments when you or your family are ill and avoid meat, fish and eggs and use no leather. (Sir Roy Calne, *Frame News*, February, 1984.)

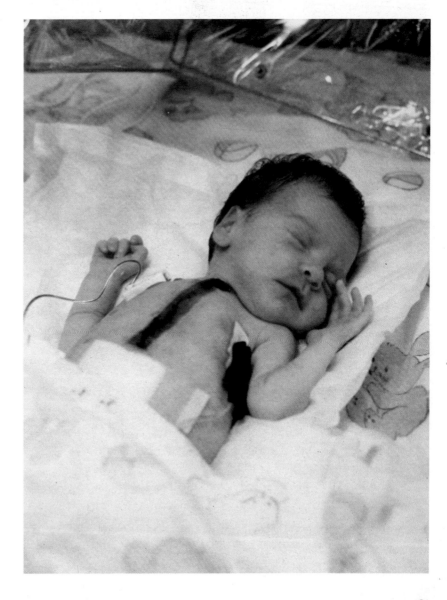

When Baby Fae was given the heart of a baboon to replace her own failing heart in 1984, a bitter debate into the ethics of such operations followed. Sadly, Baby. Fae died soon after the transplant.

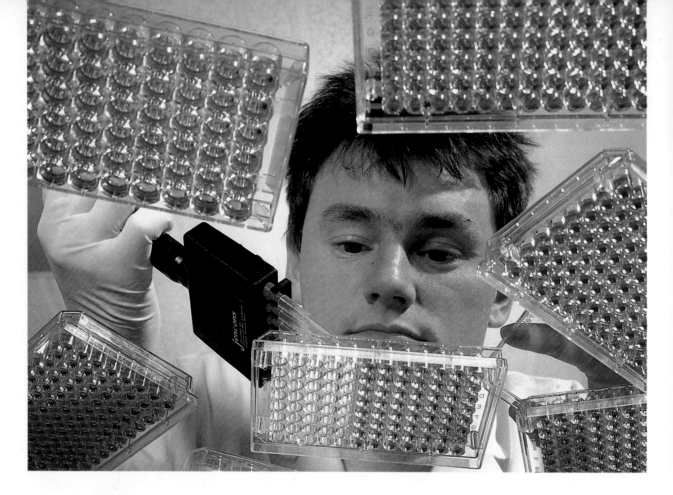

Many researchers agree that too many experiments are performed in chemical and drug testing and, indeed, the number of animals being used is falling. In addition, scientists are trying to find alternative methods of testing drugs. One method that is being used is to carry out tests on human or animal cells grown artificially in the laboratory (known as tissue cultures).

> The most immediate hope of reducing animal experiments lies in the application of better science and better experimental design, to reduce to an aboslute minimum the numbers of animals used in procedures which are justifiable and necessary, and to minimise any pain, discomfort or distress suffered.

The long term prospect of eliminating the need for live animal experiments altogether must rely on the development, validation, evaluation and adoption of reliable replacement alternative methods. (Fund for the Replacement of Animals in Medical Experiments, *Frame News,* September, 1986.)

But whether or not we 'need' to test drugs before we take them ourselves, do we have the moral right to take the lives of other species in the animal kingdom?

Above *Scientists are gradually developing alternative methods of testing new drugs which do not need animals. This scientist is working with tissue cultures.*

> As I argue, the fundamental reason why we are 'entitled' to use animals for experimentation − if we are forced to speak this way − is that they are in no sense the moral equals of humans, and therefore we are under no moral obligation to refrain from so using them. Since anything that is not prohibited by a moral imperative of some kind (that is, not morally wrong) is morally permissible, and since the use of animals for experimentation is not morally prohibited, then this use falls within that class of actions that are morally permissible. We do not need a correlative [corresponding] right to give the seal of approval to everything we do, to 'justify' it . . . (Michael Allen Fox, *The Case for Animal Experimentation,* 1986.)

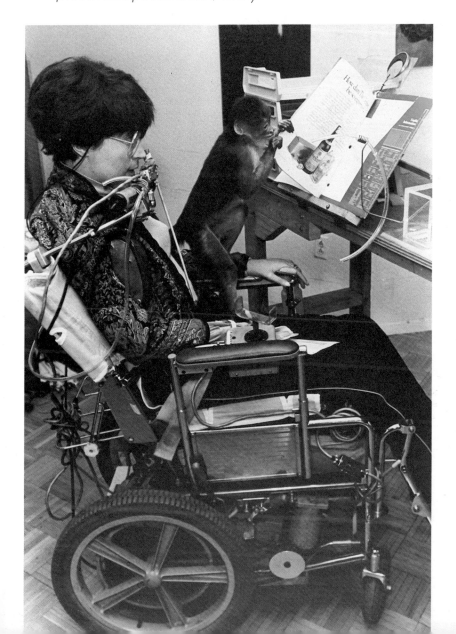

Left *Animals, like this monkey, have been trained to help the disabled by carrying out simple everyday tasks. Do we have the right to exploit animals in this way?*

Licence to experiment
Researchers cannot perform whatever experiments they like. In the UK, for example, any scientist planning to work with animals must apply to the Home Office for a licence, explaining precisely what experiments are planned. Home Office inspectors visit universities, industrial and other laboratories where research is done, to check facilities.

Animal rights supporters disagree with the idea that humans are in some way superior to animals:

> It is especially irònic that a great deal of research (such as pain studies and much psychological research) depends on the *closeness* of humans and animals rather than the reverse. There is more continuity between species than we previously thought, including the capacity to experience and suffer. Today the idea that humans are inherently superior to the other animals rings more of self assuring prejudice than of rational conclusion. (Lawrence Finsen, 'The Animal Rights People May Not Be So Misguided After All', *Los Angeles Times,* 3 June, 1985.)

As with other areas of medical ethics, animal experimentation arouses strong feelings and that can lead some people to resort to extreme and sometimes violent measures. However, you can see from reading this chapter that there are many ways of looking at the issue and arguments on all sides can be convincing. Which argument do you find most persuasive?

1 Weigh up the arguments about the rights of animals. Should the human need for better medicine be put before an animal's right to life?
2 Look at Sir Roy Calne's view about the need for animal experimentation. Does it necessarily follow that if you are an anti-vivisectionist you should also be vegetarian and avoid all animal products, including leather?
3 Do you think it is important to know how similar an animal's suffering is to our own, to decide whether or not to use it in an experiment?

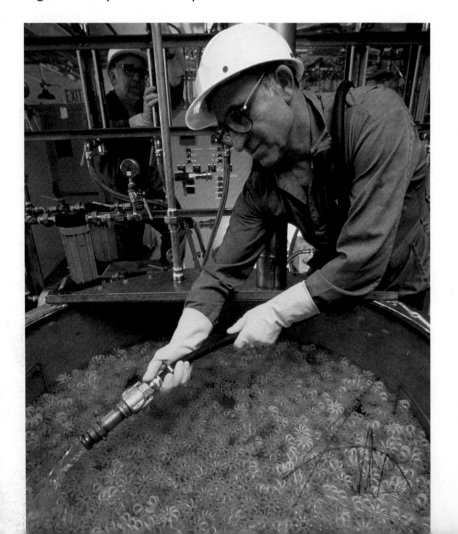

Left *Mass production of antibiotics. Should animals be used to test the effects of these and other drugs?*

5

Prevention or cure?

Wherever you live, whether there is a national health service or a system of care paid for by private insurance, cost has become a major factor influencing when, where and how disease is treated. Prevention, according to the old proverb, is better than cure. Yet, throughout the world, far more money goes into treating illness than preventing it. Why should this be?

> There is a common tendency for people to be more concerned with the concrete immediacy of the present than with the possibilities of the future . . . The successful objectives of prevention have no drama, because saved lives are non-events. (Roger Blaney, *Ethical Dilemmas in Health Promotion*.)

High-technology medicine snatches the headlines, but would the tens of thousands of pounds often spent on a single 'state of the art' heart operation be put to better use in a vaccination or cancer screening programme?

Preventive medicine in action. Here a thermogram measures variations in body heat. This can be used to diagnose breast cancer early and so prevent it spreading to other parts of the body.

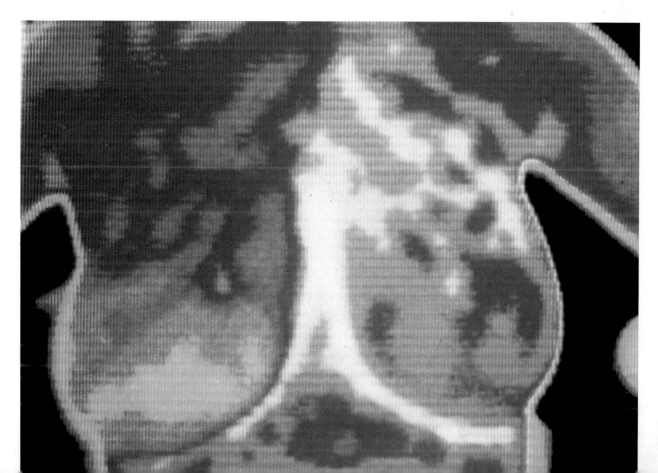

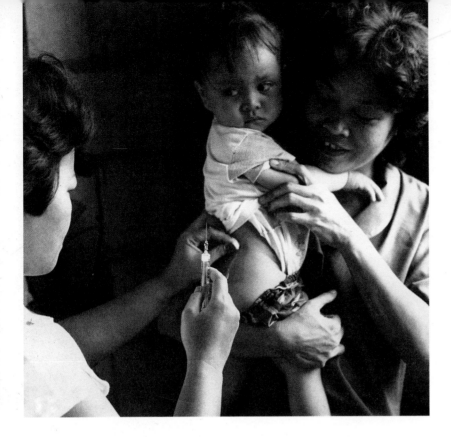

> There is no question that the amount of money being used to implant the artificial heart could improve the health of many more individuals if it were employed for preventive services. But that, and many other objections that are raised against the advance of high technology are, to me, beside the point.

Technology advances whether one agrees or not. One can turn aside or join, but as has been frequently noted, technology has its own imperative. Personally, I enjoy it. (Eric J. Cassell, *After Barney Clark,* 1984.)

And the opposing view:

> Even assuming that an artificial heart can be developed that will work well through the normal life span of a patient, how many tens or hundreds of thousands of dollars are justified in a single case of life saving? . . . [In the poorest parts of the world] the cost of a handful of heart transplants could save the sight, vigor and even the lives of thousands. (Jenkin Lloyd Jones, *Conservative Chronicle,* 10 September, 1986.)

Yet there have been significant international successes in preventive medicine. In 1980, the World Health Organization (WHO) announced the global eradication of smallpox. It was the result of a massive vaccination programme for millions of people in some of the remotest parts of the world.

The transplant revolution

Eight out of ten heart transplant patients now survive one year, and 60-70 per cent five years, after their operation. Success rates for kidney transplants are even better. Even heart-lung transplants — much newer and more difficult — are becoming increasingly successful, with three out of four patients alive and well a year after their operation.

> The eradication of smallpox, generally regarded as medicine's greatest triumph, was also an unprecedented triumph for mankind. For once, a humanitarian cause, a fight against a lethal disease captured the will of the world, uniting every country behind the leadership of WHO . . .

During the campaign, some of the world's most inhospitable landscapes were tirelessly crisscrossed by smallpox fighters, sometimes by jeep, donkey or fishing boat; sometimes — in hostile areas — under military escort, sometimes by foot in jungle or desert, journeys of up to 300 km. (WHO publicity material.)

It is a hard act to follow. WHO has set measles, whooping cough, tetanus in the newborn, polio, tuberculosis and diphtheria as targets for current mass immunization. They may not seem to be in the same killer league as smallpox, but these infections kill or cripple millions of people each year in countries where health care is not widely available.

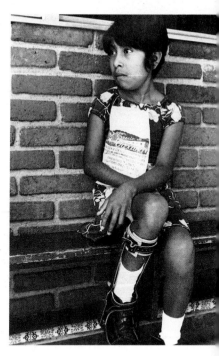

Above ·A young Mexican girl suffering from the effects of polio. Although it is now a rarity in Western countries, polio still kills or disables thousands of children in developing countries.

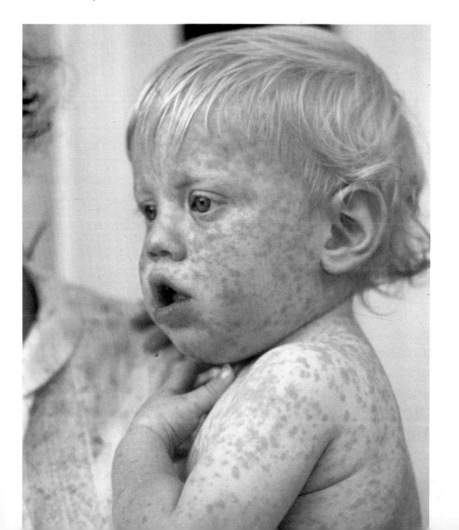

Left A baby suffering from measles — one of the many illnesses that can be prevented by immunization.

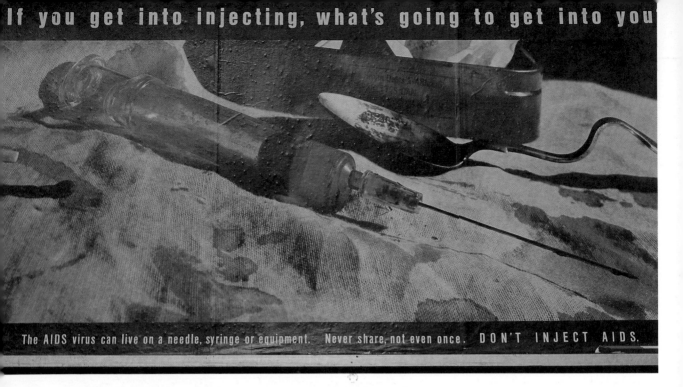

The AIDS virus can live on a needle, syringe or equipment. Never share, not even once. **DON'T INJECT AIDS.**

On top of these have come new health threats to society – AIDS and hepatitis B (see glossary). With AIDS, massive publicity campaigns in Western countries have helped to slow down the rate at which the disease is passed on. However, this was after the disease had only infected a small minority of the populations of those countries. The situation is much worse in certain developing countries, particularly in Africa. In Uganda, for example, AIDS became widespread quickly – before an effective education campaign could be launched. Now that the disease is established throughout the population, the cost of caring for those who carry the virus will put a heavy burden on the country's resources. It will also put additional pressure on the funds available for preventive medicine in Uganda.

> Most researchers agree that if no action is taken to stop the global spread of AIDS, there will be a huge disaster. Parts of Africa are already badly affected. Take the situation in Kampala, the capital of Uganda, in 1987. If a man or woman there chooses to have five sexual partners in his or her lifetime, one of them is likely to be infected with the virus . . .
> Statistics such as these are chilling. Where urban areas are so severely affected, catastrophe seems almost inevitable. (Steve Connor and Sharon Kingman, *The Search For the Virus.*)

However, some people are less pessimistic, and insist that disaster can be avoided.

Above *Striking advertisements warning drug addicts of the dangers of AIDS can now be seen in many towns and cities.*

No vaccine
There are an estimated ten million new cases of malaria each year and one million children die from the disease in Africa alone, because there is no vaccine.

Hepatitis B

Three hundred million people are carriers of hepatitis B infection – a disease which can be fatal and increases the risk of getting liver cancer by a factor of 250. There is a vaccine against hepatitis B but few developing countries, where the infection is most common, can afford it.

> Even in Africa, I'm confident in the ability of human beings to react against death. Some journalists say, 'Forget Africa. It's too late to save it.' But that's not right. If we can just show the danger to our population, I'm sure they will avoid it. No one wants to die. (Bosenge N'Galy, *Journal of the American Medical Association,* September, 1988.)

But just how effective is preventive medicine? Do health education campaigns really make people change their lifestyles to make them more healthy?

Despite all the education campaigns, at least in Western countries, an epidemic of smoking-related diseases is sweeping the world – 100,000 deaths a year in the UK, two million deaths a year in China expected by the year 2020.

> If you take 1,000 young smokers who smoke one pack a day, statistically one will be murdered, six will die on the roads, but 250 will die prematurely from smoking induced diseases . . . Today, more people are dying of an unnecessary preventable disease than died during the era of cholera. Will indifference, ignorance and vested interest continue to kill off that section of our society that cannot or will not save itself? (Duke of Gloucester, *BMA News Review,* October, 1984.)

Below *As the demand for cigarettes in Europe and the USA has diminished, manufacturers have begun a 'hard sell' in many developing countries, such as here in Papua New Guinea.*

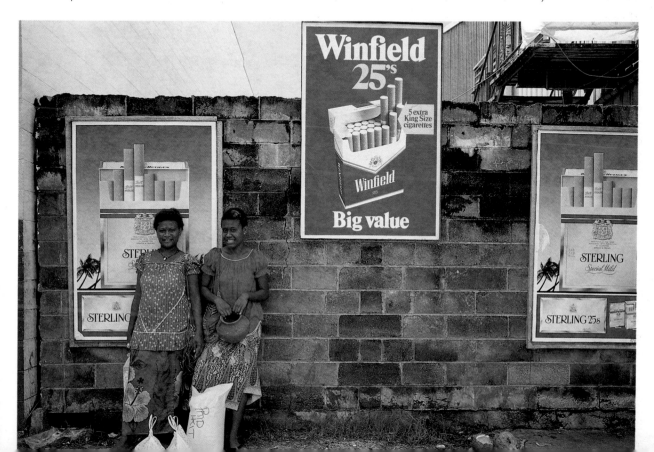

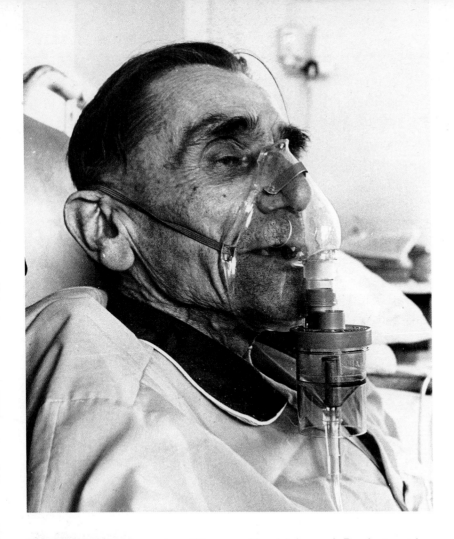

This man needs a special supply of oxygen to allow him to breathe. He has emphysema — a disease which is usually fatal. His lungs have slowly disintegrated as a result of smoking.

Nor is smoking the only self-imposed health hazard. By their mid-twenties around one in three people living in developed countries are substantially overweight, putting themselves at increased risk of heart disease, diabetes, high blood pressure and gall-bladder disease. This continues despite tremendous social pressure to be slim.

In the fight against disease, taking responsibility for our health is not always easy. But if the huge cost of curing the results of twentieth century living is to be reduced then prevention must play a greater role in health care systems.

> For many, a healthy diet may be achieved only at great cost or inconvenience and for others smoking and drinking to excess may be closely related to social pressures. Furthermore, the individual is powerless to change factors in the physical environment. Nevertheless, creating an atmosphere which would enhance the social value of prevention requires cooperative effort between the citizens and government. (Roger Blaney, *Ethical Dilemmas in Health Promotion*.)

1   Discuss the pros and cons of spending more money on preventive medicine (health education, immunization) at the expense of advances in high technology curative medicine.
2   Why do you think people are reluctant to change aspects of their lifestyle, such as smoking, diet, lack of exercise and stress, which they know are damaging their health?

6

Improving on nature?

> 'Nothing like oxygen shortage for keeping an embryo below par . . . The lower the caste,' said Mr Foster, 'the shorter the oxygen. The first organ affected was the brain. After that the skeleton. At seventy per cent of normal oxygen you got dwarfs. At less than seventy, eyeless monsters.' (Extract from the novel *Brave New World* by Aldous Huxley.)

The fictional Mr Foster describes his techniques for manipulating embryos in Huxley's novel, first published in 1932. In 1946, Aldous Huxley wrote:

> All things considered, it looks as though Utopia were far closer to us than anyone, only fifteen years ago, could have imagined. Then, I projected it six hundred years into the future. Today it seems quite possible that the horror may be upon us within a single century.

As the year 2000 approaches, are we, as Huxley predicted, approaching the era of *Brave New World?* We have, or soon will have, much of the technology needed to identify and correct genetic abnormalities. We have the means to fertilize a human egg in the laboratory *(in vitro* fertilization — IVF) and to keep it alive for days or even weeks before returning it to the mother's body (or, in a growing number of cases, a substitute mother's womb). But will society be ruled by its own technology?

In the 1977 film, Coma, *people were kidnapped and their bodies were kept in suspended animation until their organs were needed. Ten years later people were found to be selling their organs — for real!*

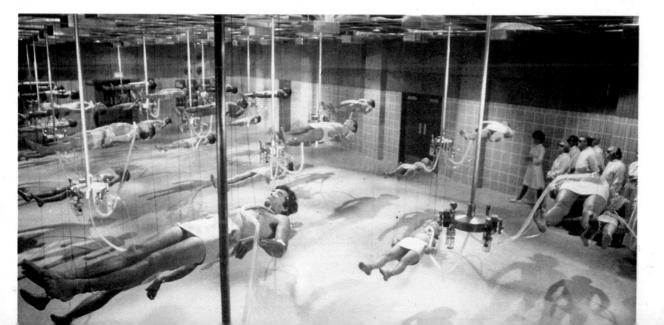

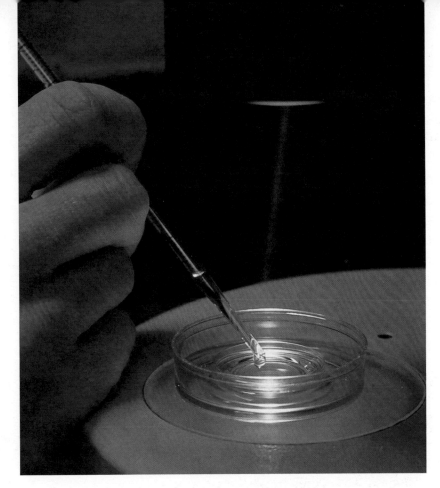

Left *The moment of conception. Human egg and sperm meet in a petri dish: so-called* in vitro *fertilization. The first test-tube baby, Louise Brown, was born in 1978.*

> Once we begin the process of human genetic engineering, there is really no logical place to stop. If diabetes, sickle cell anaemia and cancer are to be cured by altering the genetic make up of an individual, why not proceed to other 'disorders': myopia, colour blindness, left handedness? Indeed, what is to preclude a society from deciding that a certain skin colour is a disorder? . . . The question, then, is whether or not humanity should 'begin' the process of engineering future generations of human beings by technological design in the laboratory. What is the price we pay for embarking on a course whose final goal is the 'perfection' of the human species? How important is it that we eliminate all the imperfections, all the defects? What price are we willing to pay to extend our lives, to ensure our own health, to do away with all the inconveniences, the irritations, the nuisances, the infirmities, the suffering, that are so much a part of the human experience? Are we so enamoured with the idea of physical perpetuation at all costs that we are even willing to subject the human species to rigid architectural design? (Jeremy Rifkin , *Algeny,* 1983.)

Many scientists believe this is mere scaremongering, and that we are still so far away even from correcting minor genetic defects that to suggest that we are on the 'slippery slope' to producing armies of 'designer' beings is, and will remain, pure fiction.

> Overall, most of the more colourful futuristic projects often linked to IVF are still well beyond the scope of present-day science. Even should they become scientifically possible, there is every reason to expect that legislation conforming to the attitudes of the society of the day will be passed to ensure that adequate control is exercised.
> (Drs Peter Rogers and Alan Trounson, *In Vitro Fertilization Past, Present, Future.*)

Engineering cures

A number of genetically-engineered drugs are now available. These include a type of insulin (see glossary) which is less likely to cause serious allergic reactions than previous forms derived from cattle and pigs. But there have been a lot of problems with the technology, particularly in finding a way of mass-producing the product cheaply.

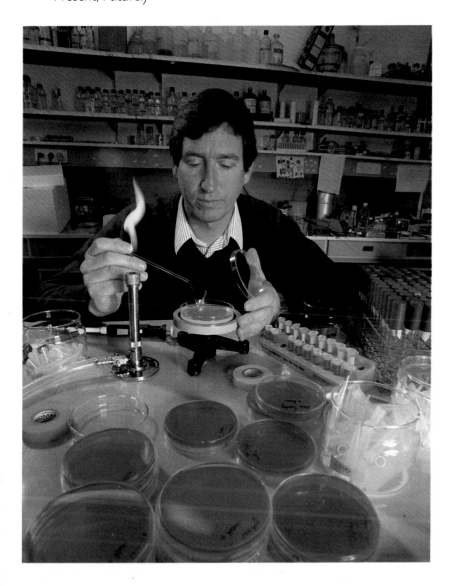

In genetic engineering, a 'foreign' gene is inserted into the genetic material (DNA) of an organism such as a bacterium or yeast.

Some governments have already taken steps to control embryo research or at least to assess the views of society.

> We accordingly recommend that no live embryo derived from *in vitro* fertilization, whether frozen or unfrozen, may be kept alive, if not transferred to a woman, beyond fourteen days after fertilization, nor may it be used as a research subject beyond fourteen days after fertilization. This fourteen day period does not include any time during which the embryo may have been frozen. We further recommend that it shall be a criminal offence to handle or to use as a research subject any live human embryo derived from *in vitro* fertilization beyond that limit. (Report of the British Committee of Inquiry in Human Fertilization and Embryology, 1984.)

Fears about genetic engineering are not restricted to its use in human patients. The technique of cutting up and transferring sections of genetic material, called DNA, is widely used for the large scale production of useful chemicals and drugs by micro-organisms such as bacteria and yeast — products which previously could be produced only in small amounts, with great difficulty or at great cost. What are the dangers of this type of genetic engineering?

Gene transplant
The first attempts to correct genetic defects were by an American scientist, Dr Martin Cline, in 1980. He attempted to correct a gene defect in two women with the blood disorder, thalassaemia, by inserting normal genes into the womens' bone marrow. The experiments failed, though they did no apparent harm. Dr Cline was severely censured for carrying out the experiments without permission from his country's regulatory bodies. No other attempts at human gene therapy have been reported.

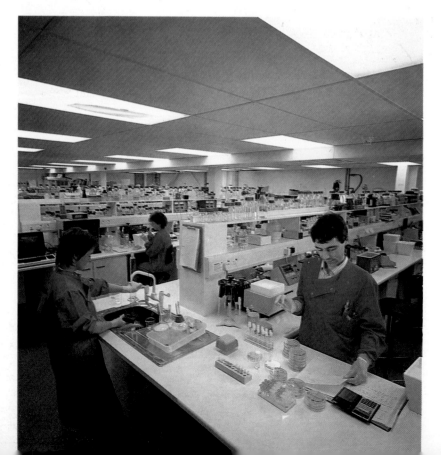

Scientists working in a modern molecular-biology laboratory. Should they be allowed to research freely, or should they be carefully controlled?

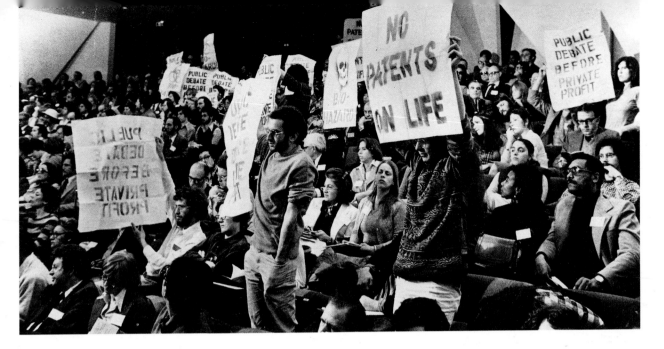

Scientists are quick to patent their discoveries so that others have to pay if they want to use them. There is now a heated debate over whether genetically-engineered organisms may be patented.

> New life forms may have dramatic potential for improving human life, whether by curing diseases, correcting genetic deficiencies or swallowing oil slicks. They may also, however, have unforeseen ramifications, and at times the cure may be worse than the original problem. New chemicals that ultimately prove to be lethal may be tightly controlled or banned, but we may not be able to 'recall' a new lifeform. (Letter to President Carter from the general secretaries of the National Council of Churches, the Synagogue Council of America and the US Catholic Conference, 20 June, 1980.)

Early in the history of genetic engineering, the Church was not alone in its fears. Leading scientists were also worried that science was moving too fast.

> . . . until the potential hazards of such recombinant DNA molecules [artificially altered genetic material] have been better evaluated or until adequate methods are developed for preventing their spread, scientists throughout the world [should] join in voluntarily deferring [postponing] . . . experiments. (Paul Berg and others, *Science* 1974, 185, 303.)

However, there were not many scientists prepared to put off what (to them at least) were critical experiments. To deal with the problem, several governments introduced regulations stipulating the type of precautions to be taken when doing experiments with varying degrees of potential risk. But, as scientists became more familiar with the new techniques, and no disasters occurred, many of the early worries began to disappear.

> Genetic engineering has now been yielding increasing benefits in medicine, agriculture and industry for six years without causing a day of illness. There is no reason to believe that the novel organisms developed for research or commerce will be more dangerous than the naturally occurring organisms from which they are derived. (Bernard Davis, *US News and World Report*, 8 October, 1984.)

This safety record has done little to convince those who were against genetic engineering in its infancy that their fears were unfounded.

> As bioengineering technology winds its way through the many passageways of life, stripping one living thing after another of its identity, replacing the original creations with technologically designed replicas, the world gradually becomes a lonelier place. From a world teeming with life, a world spontaneous, unpredictable, dynamic . . . we descend to a world stocked with living gadgets and devices, a world running smoothly, effortlessly, quietly, without feeling. (Jeremy Rifkin, *Algeny*, 1983.)

We are left with a dilemma. Is it enough that, as yet, no harm has come from genetic engineering, that the control systems in force appear to be working? Or are we being lulled into a false sense of security against which *Brave New World* could become a reality?

1 Is it right that we should attempt to correct genetic defects which may make us prone to heart disease, cancer and diabetes, or should we accept that no human being is perfect and adapt our medical services to cope with such diseases?
2 Are there any examples in history where governments have attempted to produce a 'master race'? Can you imagine society allowing the Brave New World scenario of embryos being bred for different tasks in life; with say, some 'designed' for mental excellence and others for physical prowess?
3 What other factors, besides genetics, affect the kind of adult we become?

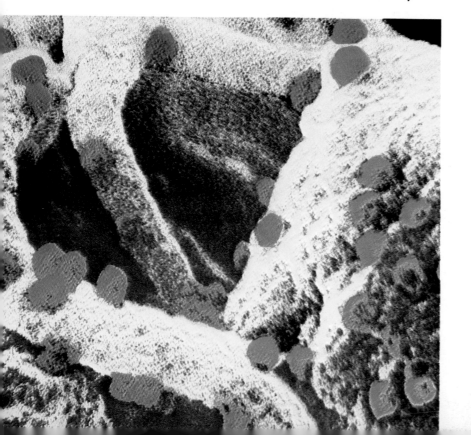

Left *A false-colour electron micrograph of the HIV virus that causes AIDS (red) budding from an infected white blood cell. Some people fear that, in the wrong hands, genetic engineering techniques might enable someone to create a virus even more deadly than HIV.*

7

World health

The World Health Organization (WHO) has set a target of 'Health for All by the Year 2000'. But there is still a huge gulf between the health care facilities of the so-called Western world and those in developing countries. Even within the better off nations there are major differences in quality of care for rich and poor, with those in the lowest social classes suffering the most illness and getting the least out of the available medical services. So how realistic is any attempt to reduce the health divide?

> Survival of the herd is perhaps the most fundamental objective of society. As life and well-being are attributes closely associated with survival, it might be concluded that their value was a 'self-evident truth'. It might be further argued that preventing pain, disability and premature death require no justification. This perspective sees life and health as either good in themselves or as desirable second level objectives.

The reality, however, is that individuals are unimportant to herd survival, and in practice the promotion of health cannot be achieved without cost, effort or resources, bringing it into conflict with competing demands, and compelling the 'value of life' to take its turn in the list of social priorities. (Roger Blaney, *Ethical Dilemmas in Health Promotion.*)

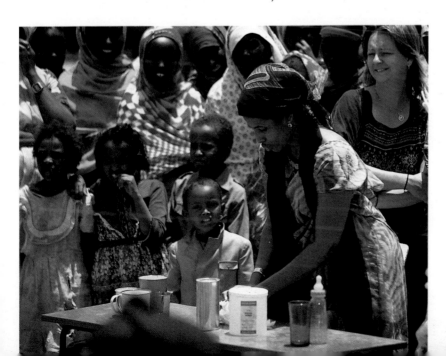

Refugees in Somalia are taught the dangers of making up infant feeds with contaminated water. Health workers try to persuade mothers to breast feed instead.

The WHO is more optimistic and believes that we can play a significant part in determining priorities for health care.

> People have the right to be involved. They need to ensure actively that their right can be given practical expression, that satisfactory prerequisites [requirements] for health exist for all, that the environment in which they live is healthy and provides conditions in which it is easy to select a healthy lifestyle, and that the health care system is responsive to their needs. It is for this reason that health for all is, above all, a movement by the people. (WHO, *Health for All by the Year 2000.*)

Yet, leaders of WHO are well aware of the obstacles to be overcome.

> There is widespread disenchantment with health care throughout the world. The reasons are not difficult to discern. Better health care could be achieved with the technical knowledge available. Unfortunately, in most countries this knowledge is not being put to the best advantage for the greatest number. Health resources are allocated mainly to sophisticated medical institutions in urban areas. . . .

A major operation in progress in a modern hospital. Even hospitals in Western countries find it hard to afford the cost of high technology surgery and medicine.

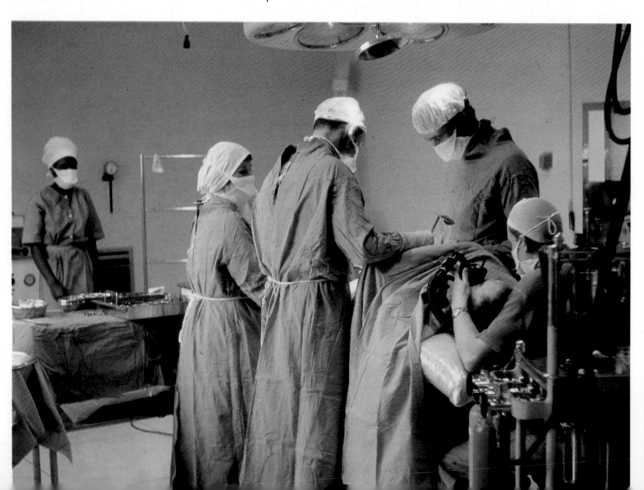

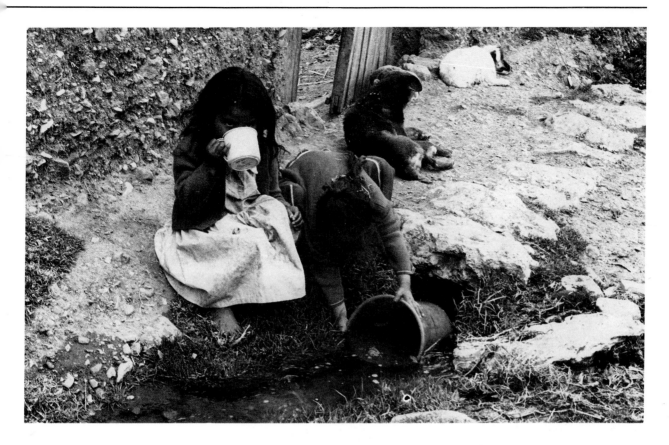

Above *Drinking unclean water is the commonest cause of illness for people in developing countries, like these children in Peru. Cholera and dysentery are just two life-threatening infections which can be caught this way.*

. . . the concentration of complex and costly technology on limited segments of the population does not even have the advantage of improving health. *(Report of WHO and UNICEF to Alma-Ata Conference on Primary Health Care, 1978* [UNICEF stands for the United Nations Children's Fund].)

The issue of priorities is crucial if standards of health care in developing countries are to improve. Governments are having to decide between spending millions of pounds on lifesaving modern drugs and high technology medical equipment, or coping with the most basic demands for clean water and better hygiene.

> There is no historical reason to expect the availability of modern drugs to transform the health prospects for those women waiting patiently, since before sunrise, in the queue for the public tap. For that listless child squatting beside the road, its life slowly draining away with its diarrhoea, the idea that some new drug, synthesized [made artificially] in a laboratory halfway around the world, will somehow help it over the multiple hurdles of malnutrition and infection to its fifth birthday is preposterous. (Mike Muller, *The Health of Nations,* 1982.)

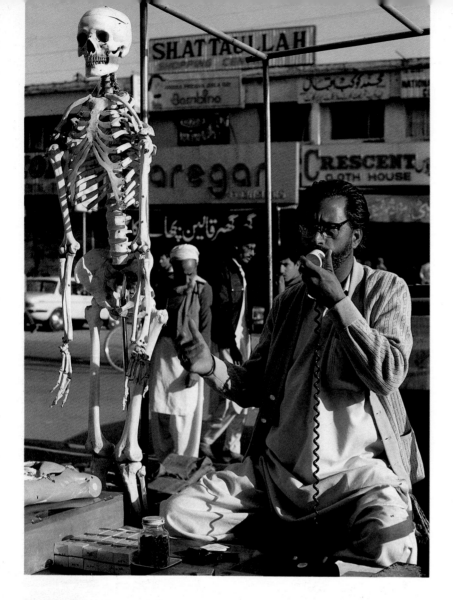

But the international pharmaceutical industry believes that medicines, alongside better nutrition and hygiene, do have an important role to play.

> Appropriate use of pharmaceutical products can provide an umbrella of protection from disease under which to tackle the fundamental causes of ill health — poverty, hunger, lack of clean water and sanitation and so on.
>
> This can usually be achieved without resorting to the latest, most expensive discoveries available. Often it is unspectacular well-known and well-tried medicines which are most desperately needed. The 'wonder drugs' of yesterday's rich world are the essential medicines of the poor world today. (Association of the British Pharmaceutical Industry, *Health in Developing Countries*.)

Health care spending expressed as a percentage of gross national product (GNP), 1984

USA	10.3%
West Germany	9.0%
Sweden	8.9%
Netherlands	8.6%
France	8.3%
UK	5.9%
Japan	5.1%

Life expectancy, 1986	
Norway	76
Australia	75
Canada	75
UK	74
USA	74
Venezuela	68
Ghana	59
India	55
Kenya	54
Mozambique	44

In 1977, the WHO produced a list for developing countries of 200 essential drugs and suggested that governments save money by avoiding other products. The pharmaceutical industry has come in for sharp criticism, over the last two decades, for the way in which it markets and promotes drugs in developing countries.

> Drugs not authorized for sale in the country of origin — or withdrawn from the market for reasons of safety or lack of efficacy — are sometimes exported and marketed in developing countries; other drugs are promoted and advertised in these countries for indications that are not approved by the regulatory agencies of the countries of origin. (Dr Halfdan Mahler, Director General of WHO, 1975.)

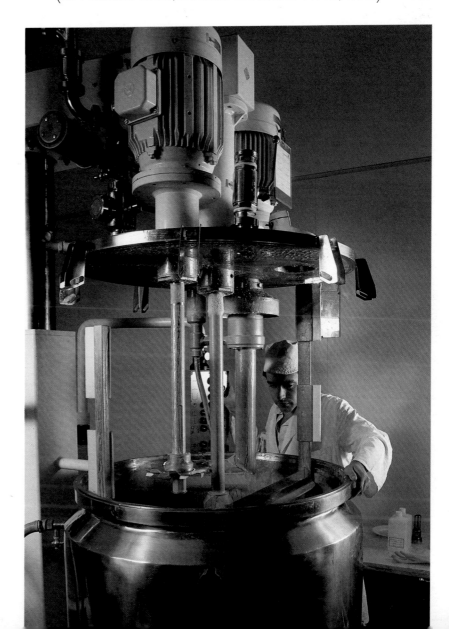

Right *Industrial manufacture of medical drugs in a modern factory in Israel. Major drug manufacturers are sometimes accused of making too much profit from ill health.*

But from the industry:

> Misinformation must be stopped, but on the whole it is the dearth of medicines, not their excessive use, which helps to perpetuate poor world health problems . . .
>
> For example, it may be suggested that when a drug is being used by a village health worker or being passed 'under the counter' to a sick person the appropriate question to ask is not 'could some people die as a result?' but, 'will more die if the drug is not available?' (Office of Health Economics, *Medicines, Health and the Poor World.*)

Inequalities in health, as already mentioned, are not limited to developing countries. In 1980 a Department of Health Working Group in the UK came to the conclusion that the health of lower-paid workers during the 1960s and 1970s, compared to that of well-paid professionals, had actually deteriorated.

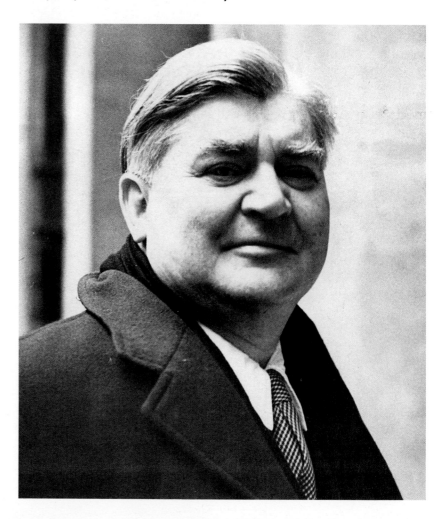

Aneurin Bevan (1897-1960), who set up the British National Health Service in 1948 so that medical care would be available 'to rich and poor alike in accordance with medical need and by no other criteria.'

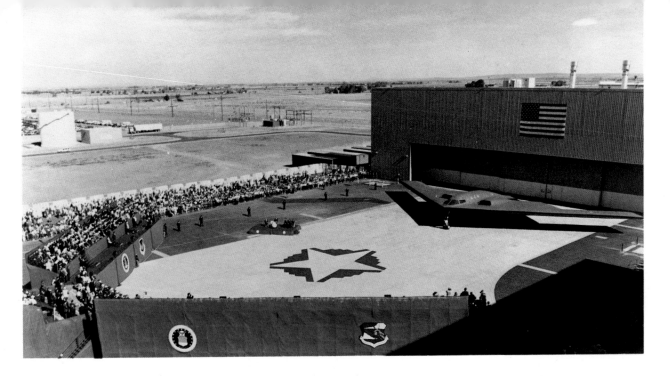

This in a country which, in 1948, set up a National Health Service (NHS) whose prime goal was to provide medical care for its people regardless of their ability to pay. The 1980 report, produced by the Department of Health Working Group, advised that to improve health care substantially, the government would have to direct much more money into the health care system. However, the government replied that the funds were simply not available:

> It will come as a disappointment to many that over long periods since the inception of the NHS there is generally little sign of health inequalities in Britain actually diminishing and, in some cases, they may be increasing . . . I must make it clear that additional expenditure on the scale which could result from the report's recommendations – the amount involved could be upwards of £2 billion a year – is quite unrealistic in present or any foreseeable economic circumstances . . .
> (Patrick Jenkin, *Inequalities in Health*, 1980.)

Rich country or poor, lack of money seems to be at the root of many of the problems of world health. There is an additional dilemma for Western countries such as the USA and those in Europe and Australasia. While the demands on medical services in developing countries are made mainly by the very young, the huge increase in numbers of elderly people in more prosperous societies looks set to stretch health care provision to breaking point. The medical needs of the elderly are expensive both in medical equipment and manpower. As yet, no country has found a solution.

Each Northrop B-2 bomber – the latest in American military equipment – costs $516 million to build. Would the money be better spent on health care, or is defence more important?

1   Why do you think there are such differences in death and illness rates between the rich and poor of the wealthier nations such as the USA and the UK?
2   Make a list of the things you would expect a government to provide; for example: education, health care, policing. Arrange the list with the most important services at the top and the least important at the bottom. How high up the list do you put health care?

8

Conclusion

There are no easy answers to any of the dilemmas discussed in this book, as the Most Reverend J. S. Habgood, Archbishop of York, says:

> It seems to me that one of the clearest lessons to be learnt from the history of medical ethics is that most of the interesting and difficult problems have no logical answers. This is not to say that ethical thinking need be unprincipled or reduced to mere expressions of opinion, but simply that the real dilemmas arise when facts are ambiguous, prognostications hazardous and principles are in conflict. A good moralist is one who has learnt to live with this uncomfortable mixture and weigh the significance of the various factors involved. (Most Reverend J. S. Habgood, *Philosophy and Practice of Medical Ethics.*)

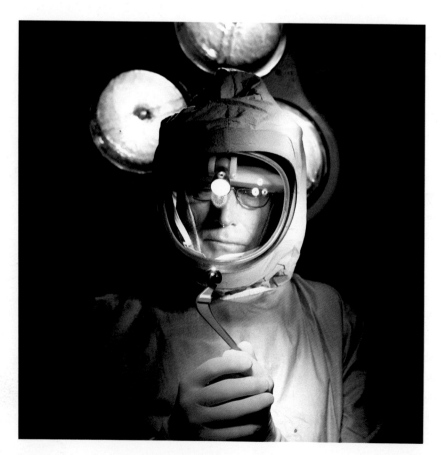

Left *This orthopaedic surgeon holds up an artificial hip joint which, when implanted, should enable the patient to walk. Despite ethical problems, medical and surgical advances have improved the quality of life of millions of people.*

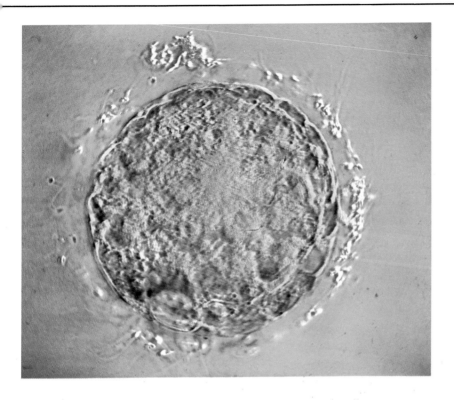

Doctors and philosophers may suggest a broad framework for the way in which ethical dilemmas should be tackled, but it is our task to ensure that any legal or moral guidelines reflect the views of society as a whole. In some cases – such as abortion and euthanasia – decisions have already been made. But these can still be changed to reflect alterations in public views of what is acceptable.

In newer areas, such as genetic engineering and other advances in medical technology, doctors and scientists are still trying to establish the boundaries within which they should be working. So here too, we must be sure that our views are heard. As a leading British philosopher points out:

> There must be some barriers that are not to be crossed, some limits fixed, beyond which people must not be allowed to go. The very existence of morality depends on it . . .
>
> . . . there will not be universal agreement about where these barriers should be placed. The question must ultimately be what kind of society can we praise and admire? In what sort of society can we live with our conscience clear? (Baroness Mary Warnock, *Report of the Committee of Inquiry into Human Fertilization and Embryology,* 1984.)

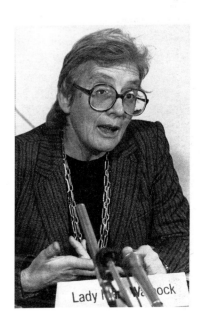

Below *Baroness Mary Warnock – leading philosopher and head of the British government committee which reported on embryo research in 1984.*

Lady Mary Warnock

Glossary

AIDS (Acquired Immune Deficiency Syndrome) An incurable disease of the immune system, probably caused by a virus known as the human immuno-deficiency virus (HIV), which leaves sufferers prone to increasingly serious and eventually fatal infections.

Chemotherapy The treatment of disease by chemical means.

Coma A state of unconsciousness like deep sleep, that can last for varying lengths of time, from hours to years.

Diabetes A disease in which sugar levels in the blood are too high, the result of a poor supply of insulin, the hormone made in the pancreas.

Diphtheria An acute contagious bacterial disease causing fever, and difficulty in breathing and swallowing.

Electroconvulsive therapy Treatment for mental illness that uses the effects of electric shocks on the patient.

Embryo The human embryo is the earliest stage of life, continuing up to the eighth week of the woman's pregnancy. From then on it is referred to as a fetus until the moment of birth, when it is referred to as an infant.

Euthanasia The deliberate putting to death of a person or animal in an easy, painless manner.

Fetus See embryo.

Genetic engineering The popular term for changing the genetic information, held in molecular form, and stored in cells, which determines the characteristics of living things. Scientifically referred to as recombinant DNA (deoxyribonucleic acid) technology.

Gynaecology The study of diseases of women. A gynaecologist deals with anything related to the womb and other female reproductive organs.

Hepatitis B A serious, life threatening viral infection of the liver.

Hormone One of the many chemical substances produced by the body that has specific effects on certain parts of the body.

Immunization The injection of a small amount of a virus, bacterium or parasite to arm the immune system against subsequent attack.

Malaria Serious infection caused by a parasite carried by female mosquitoes in certain parts of the world, such as Africa, Asia and Central and South America.

Neural Concerning the nerves and the central nervous system.

Neurosurgeon A doctor who specializes in surgery on the nervous system.

Obstetrics The medical speciality dealing with the care of pregnant women and the birth of their babies.

Paediatrician A doctor who specializes in the diagnosis and treatment of illness in children.

Pessary A device designed to be inserted into the vagina – as a support for the uterus, as a contraceptive or (see the quotation on page 4) to induce an abortion.

Polio Short for poliomyelitis, an infectious viral inflammation of the nerve cells in the grey matter of the spinal cord. Infection may result in temporary or permanent paralysis for the sufferer.

Prognostication The prediction of the outcome of something; for instance, an illness.

Protocol In science or medicine, a plan of action for research or for treatment.

Psychology The study of the mind, how it works and why people behave the way they do.

Quickening (When referring to a pregnant woman.) The stage of pregnancy when movements of the fetus have been felt. It happens at different times with male and female fetuses.

Senile dementia A mental disorder of the elderly caused by degeneration of brain tissue which leaves sufferers unable to think, concentrate or look after themselves.

Smallpox A usually fatal infectious disease.

Spina bifida A condition often apparent from birth, caused by a deformation of the spinal cord that can result in abnormal growth of the skull and paralysis.

Tuberculosis A communicable disease usually affecting the lungs.

Further information

You can contact these organizations to find out more about the issues covered in this book.

American Association for the Advancement of Science, 1333 H Street NW, Washington DC 20005, USA.

Australia and New Zealand Association for the Advancement of Science, GPO Box 873, Sydney, New South Wales, Australia 2006.

Australian Medical Association, PO Box 20, Glebe, New South Wales, Australia 2037.

British Association for the Advancement of Science, 23 Saville Row, London WI, UK.

Canadian Medical Association, PO Box 8650, Ottawa KIG 0G8, Canada.

Fund for the Replacement of Animals in Medical Experiments, Eastgate House, 34 Stoney Street, Nottingham NGI INB, UK.

The Association for the Advancement of Science in Canada, 2450 Lancaster Road, Suite 36, Ottawa KIB 5N3, Canada.

World Health Organization, Avenue Appia, 1211 Geneva 27, Switzerland.

Further reading

British Medical Association *Philosophy and Practice of Medical Ethics* (Unwin Brothers, 1988)

Bryan, Jenny *Twentieth Century Medicine* (Wayland, 1988)

Bryan, Jenny *Women History Makers: Health and Science* (Macdonald, 1988)

Dixon, Dr Bernard (ed) *Health and the Human Body* (Perseus Press, 1986)

Faulder, Carolyn *Whose Body Is It?* (Virago, 1985)

Hampton, Janie *World Health* (Wayland, 1987)

Huxley, Aldous *Brave New World* and *Brave New World Revisited* (Hogarth Press, 1984)

Medawar, Sir Peter *Advice to a Young Scientist* (Pan, 1981)

Paton, Sir William *Man and Mouse: Animals in Medical Research* (Oxford University Press, 1984)

Acknowledgements

The publishers gratefully acknowledge permission from the following to reproduce extracts from copyright material: American Association for the Advancement of Science, *Science,* 1974, 185, 303; American Medical Association, *Principles of Medical Ethics,* 1982; *British Medical Journal,* article by Dr Peter Bromwich, 28 February, 1987; Controller of Her Majesty's Stationery Office, *Report of the Working Group on Inequalities in Health,* 1980; Faber & Faber, *The Health of Nations* by Mike Muller, 1982; *Journal of the American Medical Association,* article by Bosenge N'Galy, pp 1193, 1197-1198, 2 September, 1988; *New England Journal of Medicine,* article by Franz Ingelfinger, 31 August, 1972; Oxford University Press 1) *Moral Dilemmas in Modern Medicine* by Michael Lockwood, 1986; 2) *The End of Life* by James Rachels, 1986; Penguin Books, *The Search for the Virus* by Steve Connor and Sharon Kingman, 1988; Martin Secker & Warburg, *Sex and Destiny: the Politics of Human Fertility* by Germaine Greer, 1984; The University of California Press, *The Case for Animal Experimentation* by Michael Allen Fox, 1986; Unwin Hyman, *Philosophy and Practice of Medical Ethics,* British Medical Association; *US News & World Report,* article 'Ban Experiments in Genetic Engineering?', 8 October, 1984; Virago Press, *Whose Body is it?* by Carolyn Faulder, 1985; John Wiley & Sons, *Ethical Dilemmas in Health Promotion,* edited by Spyros Doxiadis, 1987.

The publishers would like to thank the following for providing the illustrations in this book: Camera Press 20, 26, 27 (top), 30, 35 (top), 39; Chapel Studios (David Cumming) 40; Ronald Grant Archives 9; The Kobal Collection 31; Network Photographers (Sturrock) 13 (bottom); The Research House 43; Science Photo Library *Cover,* 5, 10, 12, 14, 25, 27 (bottom), 32, 36, 44, 45 (top); Topham Picture Library 8, 11 (top), 17 (top and bottom), 18 (bottom), 19, 21, 23, 42, 45 (bottom); Tropix Photo Library 4, 28, 29, 37; Wayland Picture Library 38; Zefa Picture Library 6, 7, 15, 16, 22, 24, 33, 34, 41.

Index

Page numbers in **bold** refer to illustrations